Gua Sha Mastery

Discovering Traditional Secrets for Mental, Physical, and Spiritual Transformation, Self-Healing, and Personal Growth

Marvin Bernstein

Introducing the exclusive and captivating world of Marvin Bernstein. Immerse yourself in the timeless elegance and creativity that defines our brand. Experience the unparalleled craftsmanship and attention to detail that sets us apart. Discover the essence of sophistication and style with our exquisite collection. Copyright © 2024 Marvin Bernstein

Table of Contents

Preface

Are you prepared to begin a transformative journey towards overall well-being and personal growth? Explore the fascinating world of Gua sha and uncover its incredible healing capabilities that extend far beyond just skincare. In a world filled with stress, fatigue, and imbalance, Gua sha provides a glimmer of hope—a way to restore energy, vitality, and inner peace.

Picture a life where you start your day feeling rejuvenated, invigorated, and in tune with your physical being. Imagine a moment of pure bliss as your skin radiates with a natural glow, relieving you from the weight of everyday stress. Achieving this is not a distant dream, but something you can actually attain with the incredible power of Gua sha.

Our revolutionary book, "Gua Sha Mastery: Beyond Skincare," goes beyond traditional beauty practices to reveal the profound depths of this ancient healing technique. With a rich heritage rooted in traditional Chinese medicine (TCM), we explore the wide-ranging advantages of Gua sha for overall well-being, addressing the body, mind, and soul.

What makes "Gua Sha Mastery" stand out among the many

skincare-focused books saturating the market? It's easy to understand that genuine beauty comes from within. Although traditional skincare routines may provide short-term remedies, they frequently overlook the root causes that contribute to skin problems and overall health. Our book explores a comprehensive approach, diving into the profound effects of Gua sha to tackle the underlying issues of imbalance and disharmony.

But don't simply take our word for it—come along with us on an exciting adventure of exploration and uncovering as we:

Unraveling the Secrets of Gua Sha: Explore the fascinating history and practical uses of Gua sha, as we dispel common misconceptions and shed light on its contemporary relevance.

Discover the Healing Power: Explore the benefits of Gua sha, which enhances blood flow, encourages lymphatic drainage, and relieves tension. Experience a natural healing process that rejuvenates and restores balance to your body.

Enhance Your Skill Set: Explore innovative approaches to scraping techniques, such as holographic Gua sha and specialized microsystem therapies, to access higher realms of healing and personal growth.

Embrace a Holistic Approach to Wellness: Discover the deep connection between your mind, body, and spirit. Experience the transformative power of Gua sha, which can help you cultivate emotional resilience, improve mental clarity, and nurture a profound sense of well-being.

Craft your own daily ritual with practical tips, step-by-step tutorials, and personalized self-care routines. Empower yourself to incorporate Gua sha into your life, creating a sanctuary of healing and rejuvenation wherever you go.

And that's not all—we're excited to present our second revolutionary title, "Gua Sha Mastery: Advanced Techniques for Healing and Transformation." Whether you're a seasoned practitioner or an avid enthusiast, this book provides a comprehensive exploration of Gua sha, revealing advanced techniques and specialized applications that will take your practice to the next level.

Come and immerse yourself in the fascinating realm of holographic Gua sha, delve into the intricacies of microsystem therapies, and discover the secrets to deep personal growth. If you're looking for a way to alleviate chronic pain, delve into self-discovery, or satisfy your curiosity about the incredible possibilities of Gua sha, "Gua Sha Mastery" is the perfect resource to uncover the mysteries of this ancient healing practice.

Are you prepared to begin a remarkable adventure of healing, personal growth, and uncovering your true self? Discover the incredible benefits of Gua sha and tap into your full potential now. With "Gua Sha Wellness" and "Gua Sha Mastery" as your companions, the possibilities are limitless—embark on your wellness journey today.

Introduction

Discover the immense potential of Gua Sha with "Gua Sha Mastery" by [Marvin Bernstein], the ultimate resource for unlocking advanced techniques that promote healing and personal growth. Explore the profound world of Gua sha and unlock its incredible power to transform your overall health and wellness.

Prepare to be captivated by the fascinating world of Gua sha as you delve into the depths of its intricacies in this revolutionary book. Discover a wide range of cutting-edge techniques that will elevate your practice to new heights, from holographic Gua sha to specialized microsystem therapies.

However, "Gua Sha Mastery" goes beyond being a simple guide—it serves as a roadmap to a deep and meaningful personal transformation. Whether you're looking to find relief from chronic pain, embark on a journey of self-discovery, or are intrigued by the boundless possibilities of Gua sha, this book offers a little something for everyone.

Through detailed tutorials, helpful advice, and customized self-care practices, you will discover the art of integrating

Gua sha into your everyday routine, transforming any space into a haven of restoration and renewal. Experience a soothing and revitalizing journey as you discover the incredible benefits of Gua sha. Let go of stress, tension, and fatigue as you invite balance and harmony into your mind, body, and spirit.

Are you prepared to delve into the mysteries of Gua sha and embark on a transformative journey of healing and self-discovery? Why wait? Get your hands on "Gua Sha Mastery" now and unlock the secrets of holistic wellness.

Chapter 1

Discover the wonders of Face Gua Sha!

Introducing Face Gua-Sha, the renowned scraping massage technique crafted by the ancient wisdom of Traditional Chinese Medicine. Introducing a revolutionary remedy designed exclusively for your body. Experience the incredible benefits of enhanced blood circulation, improved lymphatic flow, and the ultimate release of muscle tension. It's time to unlock a new level of well-being. Introducing the latest innovation in skincare: a much gentler version designed specifically for your delicate facial skin. Experience the transformative power of a light gliding motion tone that effortlessly lifts and smooths your skin layer, revealing a radiant and youthful complexion. Discover a stunning collection of crystal tools, featuring exquisite shapes like jade and rose quartz. Experience the gentle touch of these tools as they effortlessly glide across your skin, applying just the right amount of pressure in a soothing upward and downward motion.

Experience the ultimate solution for reducing facial puffiness and achieving a rejuvenated appearance. Our innovative technique focuses on stimulating lymphatic drainage, effectively removing excess fluid and toxins from your skin. By promoting circulation, we ensure that your skin receives a surge of fresh blood and vital nutrients, resulting in a radiant and healthy glow. Say goodbye to puffiness and hello to a revitalized complexion. Experience the gentle sensation of softly scraping your skin layer, as it works wonders to improve micro-circulation. This innovative technique effortlessly carries oxygenated bloodstream towards the dermal layers, effectively clearing congestion and revitalizing your complexion. Prepare to witness the remarkable results of stimulated cell renewal and a radiant, brightened appearance. Experience the exhilarating rush of blood as it delivers vital nutrients, promoting cell regeneration and repairing damaged tissues. This powerful process is especially beneficial for those struggling with acne or seeking to banish acne scarring. Embrace the transformative potential of this natural phenomenon.

Introducing the ultimate game-changer for your skincare regimen - a truly remarkable and effortless addition to your morning or evening routine. In just a mere 5 minutes, experience a remarkable transformation that will leave your skin visibly lifted and radiant, guaranteed with every use.

Experience the ultimate in self-care with our exquisite Gua-Sha Tools. Crafted with precision and designed for optimal results, our tools are the perfect addition to your

Step back in time to discover the ancient origins of Gua-Sha scraping tools. These remarkable tools were meticulously crafted from extraordinary materials like bones and even cow horns, showcasing the ingenuity and resourcefulness of our ancestors. Discover the fascinating world of cow horns, where vigor and communication intertwine. It is said that cow horns possess an extraordinary ability to conduct energy, allowing cows to express themselves in ways we can only imagine. Discover the captivating world of telepathic cows, where truth and myth intertwine. While the veracity of this extraordinary phenomenon remains uncertain, there is an undeniable allure to the concept. Allow yourself to be enchanted by the possibility of cows communicating through the power of thought. Embrace the wonder and let your imagination run wild with the idea of telepathic cows. Discover the wisdom of incorporating crystals into your life today. These magnificent gemstones are not only beautiful, but they are also known for their ability to emit positive energy. Experience the power of crystals for yourself.

Discover the Incredible Benefits of Gua-sha

Your Natural Beauty Introducing Gua-Sha movement, the ultimate solution for your facial skin. This incredible technique helps eliminate the lymphatic liquid that accumulates, carrying away toxins that can lead to acne and dull, irritated skin. Say goodbye to skin woes and hello to a radiant complexion!

Experience the incredible benefits of Gua-Sha:

Introducing our revolutionary product that effortlessly shades the muscles beneath your facial skin, providing unparalleled support against sagging skin.

Discover the ultimate skincare solution that not only nourishes but also hydrates your skin layer - all thanks to our innovative companies.

Experience the ultimate relaxation with our facial skin treatment. Our unique formula effectively relieves muscle stress, providing a full-body stress alleviation like no other. Drift off to sleep effortlessly as our treatment puts your body in a parasympathetic condition. Say goodbye to sleepless nights and hello to blissful slumber.

Experience the incredible benefits of our product: it's designed to boost blood flow and circulation, giving you a revitalizing and invigorating feeling like never before.

Introducing our revolutionary solution: a powerful formula that effectively targets stagnant bloodstream, a key factor in the formation of dark circles and under-eye bags. Say goodbye to tired-looking eyes and hello to a vibrant, youthful appearance.

Introducing our revolutionary product that will transform

your skin: our blemish and acne scar-fighting solution. Say goodbye to imperfections and hello to flawless skin.

Introducing our revolutionary product that goes above and beyond in the fight against lines and wrinkles. Say goodbye to aging signs and hello to a youthful complexion. Our formula not only prevents the formation of lines and wrinkles but also works tirelessly to erase existing ones. Experience the transformative power of our product and rediscover your skin's natural radiance.

Experience the transformative power of our revolutionary facial product. Say goodbye to puffiness and hello to a slimmer, more sculpted look. Discover the secret to a rejuvenated and refreshed complexion.

Experience the transformative power of our revolutionary product that instantly lifts and plumps your skin layer. Say goodbye to dull and sagging skin, and say hello to a more youthful and radiant complexion. Try it today and see the remarkable results for yourself!

Experience the ultimate skincare enhancement with our revolutionary product. Unlock the power of deep penetration and take your post-treatment routine to the next level. Our innovative formula allows serums to effortlessly reach the deepest layers of your skin, maximizing their effectiveness and delivering unparalleled results. Elevate your skincare game and indulge in the transformative benefits of our breakthrough solution.

Experience soothing relief from throat pain and headaches caused by tight muscles or fascia. Say goodbye to discomfort with our specially formulated solution.

Discover the Art of Gua-sha: Your Guide to Performing Gua-sha at the Comfort of Your Own Home

Experience the ultimate lymphatic drainage journey, starting from the depths of your throat and jaw, and gradually ascending towards the pinnacle of rejuvenation. By commencing at the lowest point, you create a seamless flow for the liquid and toxins to gracefully drain into, acting as a harmonious funnel for purification.

Discover the secret to achieving flawless skin with our revolutionary technique. By applying gentle pressure, you'll experience a remarkable transformation. Say goodbye to redness and hello to a firmer, more radiant complexion. Don't just focus on the lymph, let your skin feel the firmness it deserves. Experience the gentle pull and lifting effect with our light-weight lymphatic tools. Designed at the perfect angle of 15-20 degrees, our tools ensure a smooth and safe application on your skin. Say goodbye to stabbing yourself and hello to a rejuvenating experience.

Discover the secret to flawless skin! When it comes to your skincare routine, remember this golden rule: always scrape towards the outer sides of your facial skin. And don't forget to sweep down from the center when you're taking care of your neck. By following this technique, you ensure that your lymph drains properly into the nodes above your collarbone. Say goodbye to dull skin and hello to a radiant complexion!

Discover the Significance of the Lymphatic System!

Discover the incredible significance of your lymphatic system, which is not just important, but doubly significant, alongside your circulatory system. Discover the fascinating world of your body's circulatory system, where your heart tirelessly pumps and purifies your bloodstream. But did you know that your lymphatic system operates in a completely different way? Unlike your circulatory system, it doesn't have a built-in pump to keep things flowing smoothly. Experience the invigorating power of lymphatic flow with the perfect combination of exercise, massage therapy, and a balanced diet. Embrace the ease and convenience of this modern lifestyle to support your body's natural detoxification process.

Discover the fascinating world of the lymphatic system, a hidden gem that remained shrouded in mystery within Western culture until just a mere two decades ago. However, ancient systems of medicine, like TCM and Ayurveda, were ahead of their time, recognizing the importance of addressing stagnation when it comes to your health. Discover the untapped potential of lymphatic drainage techniques in addressing a wide range of health concerns. While the AMA has historically overlooked the impact of lymph stagnation on disease, forward-thinking countries like Germany have embraced these techniques as a powerful solution for conditions such as fibrocystic breast disease, allergies, persistent sinusitis, arthritis, eczema, coronary disease, and beyond.

Discover the telltale signs of a sluggish lymphatic system: • Imagine your body as a luxurious residence, with your blood flowing like a pristine tap and your lymphatic system acting as the efficient drains. Introducing the incredible functionality of your body: your bloodstream is in a constant state of motion, tirelessly pumping and ensuring that your valves are always in action. Introducing a common dilemma: they often find themselves venturing into uncharted territory. Introducing a groundbreaking solution for those pesky particles that just won't budge! When those larger-than-life particles in your bloodstream refuse to be eliminated by your liver, kidneys, or even your skin, fear not! Our cutting-edge technology ensures that these stubborn particles are swiftly transported through your lymphatic vessels. Experience the detrimental effects of stagnant drains, where the lack of steady movement leads to the breeding ground for disease and stagnation.

Discover the common culprits behind sluggish lymphatic circulation:

Introducing Stress - The Silent Culprit Behind Your Health Issues! Revitalize your body and enhance your overall well-being by avoiding overwork and ensuring you have ample rest periods. By doing so, you can protect and nourish your lymph, aid in the digestion of food, and support the optimal functioning of your liver organ Qi.

Introducing: Digestive Imbalances - The Culprit Behind Your Discomfort! Are you tired of feeling congested and irritated? Look no further than your gut! It turns out that inflammatory foods and poor digestion can wreak havoc on your intestinal villi, leading to discomfort and irritation. But here's the kicker: almost all of your lymph surrounds the gut through the incredible "Gut Associated Lymph Tissue" (GALT). It's time to take control of your digestive health and say goodbye to discomfort once and for all! Discover the fascinating insights I reveal later in this captivating book, where I delve into 11 extraordinary and surprisingly simple techniques that can revolutionize your digestion. Discover the secrets to achieving optimal digestion with our comprehensive guide. Uncover the four primary culprits behind poor digestion and learn effective strategies to overcome them.

Discover the impact of nutrient deficiencies, particularly iodine, on the lymphatic system. Introducing the incredible power of iodine! Say goodbye to the harmful effects of our pesticide-sprayed world and give your body the support it needs. Iodine works wonders by nurturing your lymph at a cellular level, providing you with the ultimate protection. Discover the incredible benefits of seaweed that I've outlined for you.

Unlock the full potential of your life by releasing the shackles of shame and repressed emotions. Say goodbye to blocked circulation of pleasure and embrace a life filled with joy and fulfillment. Let go of depression and experience the freedom that comes with embracing your emotions and spirituality.

Introducing the Lymphatic System: Say goodbye to inactivity! Discover the fascinating world of the lymphatic system, where you hold the power to keep things flowing. Unlike other bodily systems, the lymphatic system relies solely on your movement to function optimally. Let's dive in and explore the importance of keeping this vital system active! Discover the hidden dangers of leading an inactive lifestyle or working a desk job. Prepare to be shocked as we reveal how these seemingly harmless habits can seriously compromise your lymphatic flow.

Discover the power of diet - certain foods have the ability to either support or prevent the explosion of lymphatic energy. Experience the unfortunate consequences of consuming poorly prepared and packaged processed sugars, such as corn syrup, and white flour. These ingredients have a detrimental impact on your lymphatic system.

Introducing Face Gua-Sha, the key to unlocking the lymphatic puzzle. This incredible technique is a game-changer, especially if you struggle with chronic mucus build-up in your sinuses. Say goodbye to stagnant energy and hello to a revitalized, free-flowing system.

Discover the transformative power of enhancing lymphatic blood flow with these simple yet effective actions: • Indulge in leisurely strolls each day, especially after meals (even just ten minutes can make a difference).

Indulge in the exquisite pleasure of savoring the luscious white section of the orange! (Click here to discover more about my captivating post on this tantalizing topic).

Indulge in the vibrant allure of red-stained foods, such as pure cranberry juice, succulent blueberries, and luscious raspberries.

Introducing a revolutionary way to enhance your daily routine: the Sit Less Method. Say goodbye to the sedentary lifestyle and hello to a more active and vibrant you. With our innovative approach, you'll effortlessly reduce the amount of time you spend sitting each day. Experience the benefits of increased energy, improved posture, and a healthier lifestyle. Don't wait any longer - take the first step towards a more active and fulfilling life with the Sit Less Method. Experience the rejuvenating power of dry-brushing with just a few minutes of your time, several times a day.

Experience the Power of Face Gua-Sha - Unleash the Beauty Within

Experience a remarkable transformation in your tone with these revolutionary facial massage therapy techniques. Unlock the secrets of a person's soul with just a glance at their face. It's not just about the lines etched on their skin or the fleeting expressions they wear. No, it's so much more. Experience the transformative power of health and fitness radiating from within, as Chinese medicine reveals the profound connection between your inner well-being and your outward beauty. Discover how your face becomes a captivating canvas that reflects the vibrant state of your internal health.

Discover how our beauty routines can revolutionize your overall health. Introducing our extraordinary creator and esteemed physician, Katie, who has ingeniously distilled the essence of ancient Chinese wisdom into a collection of remarkably potent one-minute rituals. Effortlessly achieve your health and fitness goals with ease. Seamlessly integrating into your modern lifestyle, our transformative approach will leave you with a vibrant and radiant glow, ensuring a healthy and rejuvenated appearance.

Experience the Art of Transformation

Discover three iconic Chinese beauty secrets that can transform your appearance in just minutes. We have carefully curated these approaches to ensure maximum effectiveness. Discover the incredible value of a minute for each and every one of us.

Introducing the incredible trio of rejuvenation techniques:

Àn-fa (press-hold), Gua-Sha (press stroke), and Acupressure (press-turn). These ancient methods are designed to revitalize your body and restore balance. Experience the power of touch and unlock a world of wellness with these extraordinary practices.

Discover the ancient secrets of Chinese facial massage therapy, a practice that has been cherished for its rejuvenating and calming effects for countless years.

Discover the astonishing results of our groundbreaking studies, revealing that a remarkable 82% of women experienced an immediate and uplifting transformation in just a mere minute of use.

Introducing Àn-fa: The Ultimate Solution

Experience the transformative power of our revolutionary technique. Simply place the exquisite jade Beauty RestorerTM gently against your skin and feel the soothing pressure. As you press and hold, watch as swelling diminishes and lymphatic drainage is enhanced. Unlock the secret to a more radiant and rejuvenated complexion.

Introducing the revolutionary Sweetness RestorerTM - the ultimate solution for tired eyes. Experience the blissful relief as you delicately apply this magical formula around your eyes. Say goodbye to fatigue, pesky eye bags, puffiness, and even those annoying twitching eye muscles. Embrace the soothing power of Sweetness RestorerTM and let your eyes shine with renewed vitality. Discover the incredible benefits of using the jade tool to alleviate stress-related symptoms like headaches, flushing, skin conditions, and throbbing temples. Experience the soothing power of jade and say goodbye to discomfort.

Introducing Gua-Sha - the ultimate beauty secret!

Discover the transformative power of Gua-Sha, an effortless yet effective press and stroke technique that gracefully follows the natural contours of your face, as beautifully demonstrated. Discover the timeless allure of this exquisite beauty treatment, cherished and practiced for countless generations throughout the enchanting lands of Asia. Experience the remarkable power of our product, renowned for its unparalleled ability to enhance blood circulation beneath the surface of your skin. Witness the transformative effects as it nourishes your skin and boosts collagen production.

Experience a revolutionary approach to skincare. Say goodbye to ordinary creams and serums that only work on the surface. With our innovative solution, you can activate your body's natural nourishing powers to transform your skin from within. Prepare to witness a profound and meaningful transformation like never before. Discover the incredible self-massage technique that has been scientifically proven to skyrocket circulation by an astounding 100%! Experience the incredible benefits of our revolutionary product. Our formula is designed to stimulate the dermis, helping to boost collagen production. By targeting areas of stress, it effectively relaxes cosmetic muscles, giving you a rejuvenated appearance. Not only that, but it also significantly increases blood and lymphatic circulation. Discover the transformative power of our product today. Experience the transformative power of our products, resulting in a luminous, vibrant complexion that exudes vitality and well-being.

Discover the incredible power of Acupressure!

Discover the incredible power of activating the acupressure factor on your face and unlock a world of internal organ support like never before. Discover the secret of Chinese medication, where true beauty is believed to emanate from within. According to this ancient wisdom, your organs play a vital role in revealing your overall health and radiance.

Chapter 2

Discover the World of Gua-Sha: A Comprehensive Guide

Introducing the ultimate list of top-notch materials that will leave you in awe. Prepare to be amazed as we unveil the very best options for your consideration:

Experience the elegance of Bian Stone.

Discover the extraordinary power of Bian stones, the ultimate tools for Gua-sha. With their unparalleled ultrasonic pulses and exceptional frequency collection, Bian stones are believed to be the pinnacle of therapy. Experience the ancient wisdom that has been passed down for centuries by harnessing the remarkable benefits of Bian stones. Discover the ancient wisdom of Chinese medicine as revealed in the illustrious "Nei Jing." This historical masterpiece unveils a treasure trove of healing modalities, including the renowned practices of acupuncture, moxibustion, natural medication, Qigong, and the transformative Bian rock therapy. Immerse yourself in the sacred teachings of the revered Yellow Emperor, a divine figure in Chinese religious beliefs, and unlock the secrets to optimal well-being. Discover the awe-inspiring fact that Bian rock therapy actually predates the ancient practice of acupuncture.

Experience the true essence of Gua-Sha with the unparalleled authenticity of Bian rocks.

Introducing Jade - the epitome of elegance and sophistication.

Introducing Jade, the ultimate choice for Gua-sha devices. Discover the incredible power of qi energy, a force that rivals the very vitality of your own body. Discover the ultimate solution for rejuvenating treatments - it's truly perfect for healing. Step back in time to ancient China, where resourceful barefoot doctors ingeniously turned to unconventional methods. Unable to procure the luxurious traditional Gua-sha tools, they ingeniously repurposed discarded scraps from skilled jade carvers. These humble fragments became their very own Gua-sha tools, embodying the spirit of innovation and adaptability.

Discover the timeless power of jade, still revered and widely used today for its incredible healing properties.

Introducing the exquisite Buffalo Horn!

Discover the authentic beauty of Bian rocks, sourced exclusively from the enchanting city of Sibin in China. Looking for an alternative to Bian rocks? Look no further than Buffalo horn - a truly exceptional choice.

Discover the fascinating world of Chinese medicine, where the buffalo horn is renowned for its unique combination of a refreshing coolness and a delightful acrid/salty flavor. Experience the incredible power of acridity as it enhances the flow of qi and blood circulation, providing nourishment and moisture like never before. Experience the exquisite balance of flavors as the saltiness delicately soothes, while simultaneously releasing tension and transforming hardness into a gentle tenderness. Introducing the incredible power of coldness, the ultimate solution to dispel warmth and eliminate harmful toxins from your body.

Introducing the magnificent American buffalo, no longer

on the endangered list! But if you find yourself concerned about the origin of buffalo horns, we have a stylish solution for you. Opt for exquisite jade, natural stone, or sleek steel alternatives instead.

Introducing the revolutionary Stainless Steel tools! Crafted with medical-grade precision, these tools are the top choice for DASCM (Device Assisted Soft Cells Mobilization). They represent the cutting-edge evolution of Gua-Sha techniques, bringing you the latest advancements in the field. Discover the unparalleled quality of Stainless and Titanium implements for a truly cutting-edge experience. Upgrade to these innovative materials and elevate your tools to the next level.

Introducing Rose Quartz - the epitome of elegance and beauty.

Discover the incredible power of rose quartz, renowned for its ability to unlock the heart chakra and alleviate the burdens of stress and tension in the body. Discover the exquisite charm of a delightful stone, delicately adorned in a captivating shade of red.

Experience the unparalleled smoothness and exquisite weight of our Gua-Sha tool. Discover the exquisite challenge of carrying and selecting the magnificent buffalo horn or bian rock. Some may argue that it's no easy feat, but for those who appreciate the artistry and craftsmanship, it's a testament to the dedication and skill required. Discover the versatility of Gua-Sha, where any ordinary object - whether it's a coin, a spoon, or even a simple cover - can be transformed into a powerful tool for ultimate relaxation and rejuvenation. Experience convenience and create unforgettable memories by acquiring the finest materials. With the right techniques and special tools that become uniquely yours, elevate your experience to the next level.

Experience a transformative journey towards managing your stress and diseases with the power of natural remedies. Say goodbye to relying on pharmaceuticals or fleeting vices that offer only temporary relief. Embrace a holistic approach that brings long-lasting alleviation and restores your well-being.

Experience the ultimate in self-care with our exquisite

Gua-Sha Jade Stone. Crafted with precision and care, this luxurious beauty tool is designed to enhance your skincare routine and promote a radiant complexion. Made

Discover the incredible benefits of Gua-Sha for your facial skin and neck, often referred to as the Eastern Botox or Eastern Facelift. Experience the rejuvenating power of this ancient technique. Experience the incredible results of this revolutionary Traditional Chinese Medication treatment when applied to your facial skin.

Revitalize your sagging face muscles with the help of top-notch companies.

Experience the transformative power of our revolutionary skincare product. Our formula is expertly designed to smooth and rejuvenate your skin, effortlessly reducing the appearance of lines and wrinkles. Say goodbye to dull, tired-looking skin and hello to a radiant, youthful complexion.

Discover the ultimate solution to your skincare concerns

with our revolutionary product. Say goodbye to dark circles and under-eye bags caused by the passage of time. Experience the transformation as age spots and skin discolorations fade away, revealing a rosier and more radiant complexion. Our powerful formula also works wonders in combating acne, rosacea, and other skin conditions, leaving your face flawlessly beautiful. Embrace the confidence that comes with flawless skin.

Discover the ultimate guide on how to effortlessly utilize:

Introducing our exquisite Rose Quartz Gua-Sha tools, meticulously crafted to elevate your self-care routine. Each set comes complete with a beautifully designed beginner's guide, ensuring that you unlock the full potential of this ancient beauty ritual in the comfort of your own home.

Introducing the Konjac Face Sponge - Pure, the ultimate skincare tool for a flawless complexion.

Introducing the incredible 100% Pure Konjac Sponge - the ultimate solution for all your skincare needs. This remarkable sponge not only deeply cleanses your skin, but also works wonders in eliminating stubborn blackheads and providing a gentle exfoliation experience. Say goodbye to dull and lackluster skin, and say hello to a radiant and rejuvenated complexion. Try the Pure Konjac Sponge today and experience the transformative power of this skincare essential. Introducing the groundbreaking online like framework powered by the incredible veggie fibers. Experience the invigorating effects of enhanced blood flow and rejuvenated skin cell renewal.

Introducing the foolproof guide to using our incredible product: Step 1: Prepare for success by giving the sponge a thorough wash. Discover the ultimate solution for maximum effectiveness: immerse it in refreshing, ordinary water and gently compress it at regular intervals. Experience the ultimate comfort for your skin with our revolutionary sponge. Before use, simply ensure that the sponge is fully hydrated, allowing it to absorb water completely. This ensures a luxurious and moisturizing experience like no other.

Indulge in a gentle and soothing massage, delicately

caressing your facial skin and body with a luxurious circular motion. Experience the transformative power as it exfoliates away dull and lifeless skin cells, revealing a radiant and deeply cleansed complexion. Experience the invigorating power of our massage, designed to revitalize tired skin and promote a youthful glow through enhanced skin renewal. Elevate your cleaning routine with our innovative sponge. Designed to perfection, it effortlessly tackles dirt and grime. And here's the best part - you have the option to infuse it with your favorite soap or cleansing solution for an even more refreshing experience. Although not essential, it's the little touch that takes your cleaning game to the next level.

Introducing the ultimate sponge that stands the test of time! With a lifespan of nearly a year, our exceptional sponge is built to endure. However, when it starts to show signs of wear and tear, it's time to bid farewell and welcome a fresh, revitalized sponge into your life. Upgrade your current item with a brand new replacement. Discover the secret to prolonging the lifespan of your sponge: give it the care it deserves.

Introducing the Konjac Face Sponge - Bamboo Charcoal,
the ultimate skincare tool for a radiant complexion.

Experience the ultimate cleansing power with the Konjac Sponge infused with Bamboo Charcoal. This incredible sponge is packed with nutrient-rich activated carbon, working tirelessly to deeply cleanse your pores and banish blackheads, dirt, and grime. Not only that, but it also effortlessly absorbs excess oils and toxins, leaving your skin feeling refreshed and revitalized. Say goodbye to clogged pores and hello to a radiant complexion! Introducing our revolutionary all-natural antioxidant that not only eliminates persistent acne-causing bacteria, but also provides an efficient and natural treatment for acne. Say goodbye to stubborn breakouts and hello to clear, radiant skin!

Unlock the full potential with our step-by-step guide on how to use our product:

Experience the ultimate cleanliness with our sponge by giving it a thorough wash before use. Experience the ultimate solution for your needs - immerse it in refreshing, ordinary water and indulge in the satisfaction of frequent, invigorating squeezes. Experience the ultimate hydration with our revolutionary sponge. Before indulging in its luxurious touch, ensure maximum moisture by allowing it to fully absorb water. Your skin deserves nothing less than perfection.

Experience the ultimate in skincare with our revolutionary technique of gently massaging your facial skin and body in a luxurious circular motion. This exquisite method not only exfoliates dead skin cells but also deeply cleanses, leaving your skin feeling rejuvenated and radiant. Experience the invigorating power of our massage, designed to revitalize tired skin and promote a youthful glow. Discover the rejuvenating benefits of stimulating your exhausted epidermis and unlocking its natural renewal process. Elevate your cleaning routine with our versatile sponge. Designed to effortlessly remove dirt and grime, this sponge is a must-have for any household. For an extra touch of freshness, you can add your favorite soap or cleansing solution, although it's not necessary. Experience the ultimate cleaning experience with our exceptional sponge.

Introducing the incredible longevity of our sponge - a true game-changer for your cleaning routine! With a lifespan of nearly a year, this remarkable sponge is built to withstand the test of time. However, should you notice any signs of wear and tear or a decline in performance, it's time to bid farewell to your trusted companion. Upgrade your current item with a brand new replacement. Discover the secret to prolonging the lifespan of your sponge with proper care.

Introducing the incredible Konjac Face Sponge in the refreshing Green Tea Herb variant!

Introducing the incredible Green Tea Extract Herb! Bursting with natural antioxidants, this powerful herb is here to revolutionize your skincare routine. With its cell-protecting function, it delivers a remarkable antioxidant impact that shields your precious skin from the harmful effects of free radicals. Say goodbye to dull and damaged skin, and say hello to a radiant and youthful complexion! Introducing our incredible natural component that works wonders for your skin! Experience the softening and plumping effects that enhance elasticity and refresh your skin's appearance. Perfect for those who want to shield their skin from the signs of aging.

Unlock the full potential with our step-by-step guide on how to use our product:

Experience the ultimate cleanliness with our revolutionary sponge. Prior to use, indulge in the ritual of thorough washing. Embrace the feeling of pristine hygiene as you prepare to embark on your cleaning journey. Experience the ultimate freshness by immersing it in refreshing water and gently squeezing it at regular intervals. Experience the ultimate comfort and care for your skin with our exceptional sponge. To ensure maximum effectiveness, simply allow the sponge to fully absorb water before delicately placing it against your skin layer. Embrace the luxurious sensation and indulge in a truly rejuvenating experience.

Indulge in the gentle art of massaging your facial skin and body, using a soothing circular motion. Experience the transformative power of exfoliating away dull, lifeless skin cells and achieving a deep, rejuvenating cleanse. Experience the invigorating power of our massage, designed to revitalize tired skin and promote a youthful glow through enhanced skin renewal. Elevate your cleaning routine with our innovative sponge. Designed to perfection, this versatile tool allows you to effortlessly apply soap or cleansing solution for an enhanced cleaning experience. While it's not essential, the choice is yours to indulge in a truly luxurious clean. Experience the difference today!

Introducing the ultimate sponge that stands the test of time! With an impressive lifespan of nearly a year, our sponge is built to endure. However, when it starts to show signs of wear and tear, it's time to bid farewell and welcome a fresh, rejuvenating replacement. Upgrade your current item with a brand new replacement. Discover the secret to prolonging the lifespan of your sponge with our superior treatment methods.

Introducing the Konjac Face Sponge - a skincare essential loved by beauty enthusiasts all the way from France! Introducing the exquisite Pink Clay!

Introducing the perfect Konjac Sponge, designed to combat the harsh effects of air conditioning, excessive sun exposure, and central heating. Say goodbye to dry, dull skin and hello to a revitalized, radiant complexion. Experience the exquisite benefits of Pure French Red Clay. This luxurious clay gently purifies, leaving your delicate epidermis feeling refreshed and rejuvenated. Not only does it effectively cleanse, but it also works wonders on boosting elasticity, giving your skin a softening and plumping effect. Discover the secret to a more radiant and youthful complexion with our Pure French Red Clay.

Discover the ultimate guide on how to use our incredible product: Step 1: Prepare for perfection by washing the sponge thoroughly before use. Discover the ultimate solution for maximum effectiveness: immerse it in refreshing, ordinary water and gently squeeze it at regular intervals. Experience the ultimate comfort with our premium sponge. Before indulging in its softness against your skin, ensure it is fully hydrated. Allow it to absorb water completely, ensuring a luxurious and refreshing experience.

Indulge in a gentle and soothing massage, delicately caressing your facial skin and body in a mesmerizing circular motion. Experience the transformative power as it exfoliates away dull and lifeless skin cells, revealing a radiant and deeply cleansed complexion. Experience the invigorating power of our massage, designed to revitalize tired skin and promote a youthful glow through enhanced skin renewal. Elevate your cleaning routine with our versatile sponge. Designed to effortlessly remove dirt and grime, this sponge is a must-have for any household. For an extra touch of freshness, simply add your favorite soap or cleansing solution. While not essential, it will take your cleaning experience to the next level. Upgrade your cleaning game with our innovative sponge today!

Introducing the ultimate sponge that stands the test of time! With a lifespan of nearly a year, our remarkable sponge is built to endure. However, when it starts to show signs of wear and tear, it's time to bid farewell and welcome a fresh replacement. Upgrade your current item with a brand new replacement. Discover the secret to prolonging the lifespan of your sponge with proper care and maintenance.

Introducing the Konjac Face Sponge in Lavender! Experience the power of lavender, an all-natural relaxant and detoxifier, with impressive healing properties. Treat yourself to the ultimate skincare experience. Introducing the exquisite beauty of this magnificent blossom, whose remarkable abilities to relax and alleviate stress and anxious tension make it the ultimate choice for indulgent and soothing skin treatments.

Discover the ultimate guide on how to use our incredible product! To ensure optimal results, it is essential to start by thoroughly washing the sponge. This simple yet crucial step will guarantee a flawless experience like no other. Experience the ultimate solution for your needs by immersing it in refreshing, ordinary water and gently compressing it at regular intervals. Experience the ultimate comfort for your skin with our premium sponge. Before use, ensure maximum hydration by allowing it to fully absorb water. Your skin deserves nothing but the best.

Indulge in a gentle and soothing massage, delicately caressing your facial skin and body in a mesmerizing circular motion. Experience the transformative power as it exfoliates away dull and lifeless skin cells, leaving you with a deeply cleansed and rejuvenated complexion. Experience the invigorating power of our massage, designed to revitalize tired skin and promote a youthful glow through skin renewal. Elevate your cleaning routine with our versatile sponge. While it's not essential, you have the option to infuse it with your favorite soap or cleansing solution for an extra refreshing experience.

Introducing the ultimate sponge that stands the test of time! With a lifespan of nearly a year, our remarkable sponge is built to endure. However, when it starts to show signs of wear and tear or loses its luster, it's time for an upgrade. Upgrade your current item with a brand new replacement. Discover the secret to prolonging the lifespan of your sponge with proper care and maintenance.

Discover the Incredible Benefits of Gua-Sha!

Introducing the incredible power of Gua-sha! This ancient technique has been known to work wonders in reducing swelling, making it the go-to solution for tackling chronic pain caused by ailments like arthritis and fibromyalgia. Not only that, but it also works its magic on muscle and joint pain, providing much-needed relief. Experience the transformative effects of Gua-sha today!

Discover the incredible potential of Gua-sha, a technique that may offer relief from a variety of conditions, including:

Introducing Hepatitis B: The Ultimate Guide to Understanding and Overcoming this Silent Threat

Introducing Hepatitis B - the viral infection that ignites liver inflammation, inflicts liver damage, and leaves behind lasting liver scarring. Discover the incredible benefits of Gua-sha, backed by scientific research, that can help you effectively reduce persistent liver inflammation.

Discover the remarkable findings of a renowned research study that meticulously tracked the journey of a man grappling with elevated liver enzymes, a telltale indication of liver irritation. Experience the incredible benefits of Gua-sha medication! Witness the remarkable results within just 48 hours of treatment as liver enzymes are significantly reduced. Don't miss out on this life-changing opportunity! Discover the incredible potential of Gua-sha! Not only is it known for its numerous benefits, but some experts even suggest that it can effectively aid against liver swelling. By doing so, it may help reduce the risk of liver harm. Experience the power of Gua-sha today! Discover the exciting world of ongoing research.

Experience the relief you've been searching for with our revolutionary solution for migraine headaches.

Experience relentless migraines even after trying multiple "over-the-counter medications"? Discover the potential relief of Gua-sha. Discover the incredible power of Gua-sha, an ancient curing technique that has the potential to provide relief for chronic headaches. According to a report from a reliable source, a 72-year-old female suffering from persistent migraines experienced remarkable results after receiving Gua-sha treatments for just 2 weeks. This remarkable success story suggests that Gua-sha could be the efficient fix you've been searching for. Say goodbye to your headaches and embrace the healing power of Gua-sha today!

Experience the discomfort of breast engorgement no more!

Experience the common issue of breast engorgement that many breastfeeding women face. Discover the discomfort caused by an overfilled chest, typically occurring in the initial weeks of breastfeeding. Experience the unfortunate discomfort of an inflamed and painful mother's breast, making it challenging for precious little ones to latch on.

Discover the secret behind this temporary setback.

Discover the incredible benefits of Gua-sha for women during their entire journey from pregnancy to postpartum. According to a groundbreaking study, women can now receive Gua-sha treatments starting from the very next day after expecting and continue enjoying its rejuvenating effects until they depart from a healthcare facility. Experience the soothing and revitalizing power of Gua-sha throughout your entire maternity experience. Introducing the revolutionary gua-sha medication for women during the postpartum period! Experience the incredible relief from engorgement, including the discomfort of fullness and pain in your breasts. Say goodbye to breastfeeding challenges and embrace the ease and joy it brings. Join the countless women who have found solace and convenience with gua-sha. Make breastfeeding a breeze with our innovative solution!

Experience the ultimate relief from neck pain.

Introducing the incredible Gua-sha technique - the ultimate solution for chronic throat pain. Discover the incredible power of this therapy as 48 research participants were carefully divided into two groups. Experience the power of gua-sha or the soothing relief of a thermal heat pad to effectively combat throat pain. Choose your preferred method and say goodbye to discomfort. Experience the incredible benefits of gua-sha! In just one week, those who were lucky enough to receive gua-sha treatment reported a significant reduction in pain. Don't miss out on this amazing opportunity to alleviate your discomfort!

Discover the fascinating world of Tourette syndrome!

Experience the undeniable signs of Tourette's syndrome, where involuntary movements like face tics, neck clearing, and vocal outbursts take center stage. Embrace the unique characteristics that define a person with Tourette's. Experience the powerful benefits of Gua-sha, combined with a range of other therapeutic techniques, to potentially alleviate symptoms of Tourette's syndrome. Discover how this innovative approach may bring relief to those seeking relief from the challenges of Tourette's.

Introducing the remarkable case of a 33-year-old male who bravely battled Tourette syndrome since the tender age of 9. Seeking relief, he embarked on a transformative journey that included the ancient art of acupuncture, the power of natural herbs, the rejuvenating practice of gua-sha, and a complete overhaul of his lifestyle. The results? Astounding. Witness his symptoms alleviated by an impressive 70 percent, paving the way for a brighter, more fulfilling life. Discover the undeniable importance of further research, even in the face of a positive test result.

Experience the relief you deserve with our revolutionary solution for premenopausal syndrome.

Experience the transformative phase of pre-menopause, a natural occurrence that takes place in women as they approach menopause. Introducing our revolutionary solution for those sleepless nights:

- Insomnia, the ultimate symptom that keeps you tossing and turning. Say goodbye to counting sheep and hello to a restful slumber. Experience the relief you've been longing for with our innovative

- Experience the freedom of a regular menstrual cycle.

- Introducing: Anxiety.

- Experience the ultimate energy drain with our revolutionary Fatigue solution.

- Experience the sizzling sensation of hot flashes!

Discover the remarkable findings of studies indicating that gua-sha has the potential to alleviate premenopausal symptoms in select women. Discover the groundbreaking analysis that delved into the lives of 80 remarkable women, each grappling with the challenges of premenopausal symptoms. Experience the transformative power of our cutting-edge procedure group. Indulge in 15 luxurious and invigorating tiny gua-sha treatments, carefully curated to rejuvenate your body and mind. Immerse yourself in the ultimate wellness journey as you receive these treatments once weekly, accompanied by our exceptional standard therapy. Prepare to be amazed as you embark on an eight-week voyage towards optimal well-being. Experience the power of regular therapy with our exclusive control group.

Experience the remarkable results of our analysis. The involvement group has reported a significant reduction in symptoms such as insomnia, anxiety, exhaustion, headaches, and hot flashes. Compared to the control group, our findings show an impressive increase in relief. Say goodbye to sleepless nights, overwhelming stress, and debilitating headaches. Trust in our research-backed solution to bring you the relief you deserve.

Discover the incredible potential of gua-sha therapy, a safe and effective treatment that experts highly recommend for alleviating these troublesome symptoms.

Discover the Truth: Unveiling the Potential Side Effects of Gua-sha

Discover the incredible benefits of gua-sha, the ultimate

all-natural healing treatment that is not only effective but also completely safe. Experience a transformative skincare treatment that may enhance the appearance of your skin. Our procedure involves gentle massaging and scraping of the epidermis using a specialized massage therapy tool. While it is not reported to be unpleasant, it's important to note that this technique may cause a temporary change in the look of your skin. Due to the delicate nature of the procedure, there is a possibility that tiny blood vessels called capillaries near the surface of your skin may burst, resulting in minimal bruising and minor blood loss. Say goodbye to unsightly bruises in just a matter of days!

Discover the incredible effects of gua-sha treatment, where many individuals also enjoy the temporary indentation of their skin.

Introducing the three indispensable precautions that must be taken:

Experience the ultimate in safety and hygiene with gua-sha therapy. Our highly skilled technicians take every precaution to ensure your well-being. In the unlikely event of any bleeding, rest assured that our tools are meticulously disinfected after each and every person. Your health and safety are our top priorities.

Discover the secret to achieving optimal results by steering clear of this technique if you've recently undergone any surgery within the last six weeks.

Discover the exclusive benefits of gua-sha, a rejuvenating practice that promotes overall well-being. Please note that individuals who are currently taking bloodstream thinners or have clotting disorders may not be suitable candidates for this invigorating treatment.

Chapter 3

Discover the incredible uses of Gua-sha!

Unveiling a multitude of ways to experience the transformative power of the gua-sha meditation technique:

Introducing Gua-sha, the ultimate solution for soothing muscle and joint pain. Introducing the remarkable world of musculoskeletal disorders! These intricate complications arising from the muscles and bone tissue are nothing short of fascinating. Prepare to be amazed by a myriad of examples, including the ever-persistent back pain, the relentless tendon stress, and the notorious carpal tunnel symptoms. Brace yourself for a journey into the captivating realm of musculoskeletal disorders!

Discover the incredible benefits of gua-sha! Not only does this ancient practice help fight disease, but it also reduces irritation. Experience the power of gua-sha today! Discover the incredible benefits of gua-sha, a powerful technique that can help you effectively address chills, fevers, and even respiratory issues. Experience the soothing and healing effects of gua-sha today!

Introducing the all-new and improved "•"! This revolutionary product is here to change the game. With its sleek design Introducing micro-trauma, the small injuries that can occur to the body, such as those resulting from gua-sha, leaving behind nothing but mere bruises. Discover the incredible power of these revolutionary products that can provide a solution to the problem of scar tissue formation. Experience the amazing results as they work their magic on your body, delivering a reply that can help separate and diminish the appearance of scar tissue. Say goodbye to unwanted scars with these remarkable products! Introducing micro-trauma, the secret weapon against fibrosis! Say goodbye to the excessive accumulation of connective tissue during the healing process. Experience the power of micro-trauma today!

Introducing the all-new and improved

•Introducing the revolutionary technique used by skilled physiotherapists - IASTM! Say goodbye to connective tissues that refuse to budge those stubborn bones. Whether it's caused by repetitive stress damage or any other condition, IASTM is here to save the day! Discover the incredible benefits of incorporating Gua-sha into your wellness routine. Enhance your results by combining this ancient technique with other complementary treatments, like extending and conditioning exercises. Unleash the full potential of your self-care journey and experience the transformative power of Gua-sha.

Discover the Amazing Benefits of Gua-Sha

Discover the groundbreaking research conducted on a new group of individuals to unveil the incredible benefits of gua-sha. Introducing the incredible lineup of products:

Experience the beauty of women near menopause.

Introducing the revolutionary Guitar Neck, the ultimate solution to alleviate discomfort caused by prolonged computer use. Say goodbye to pain and hello to productivity with this innovative accessory. Experience the perfect harmony between comfort and efficiency. Get your Guitar Neck today and start playing your way to a pain-free work experience!

Introducing our revolutionary product designed specifically for male weightlifters: the ultimate solution to enhance recovery after intense training sessions.

Introducing a solution for the aches and pains that come with age - our revolutionary product designed specifically for older adults experiencing back pain.

Discover the incredible benefits of gua-sha! Women experiencing bothersome pre-menopausal symptoms like perspiration, insomnia, and headaches have reported a significant reduction in these discomforts after incorporating gua-sha into their routine. Say goodbye to those pesky symptoms and embrace a more balanced and rejuvenated you with gua-sha!

Discover the incredible benefits of gua-sha! According to a groundbreaking 2014 study, this ancient technique has been shown to enhance motion and alleviate pain in individuals who spend long hours on personal computers. Say goodbye to discomfort and unlock a world of relief with gua-sha! Discover the remarkable benefits of gua-sha therapy for weightlifters. In a groundbreaking study conducted in 2017, it was revealed that weightlifters who underwent gua-sha therapy experienced a significant improvement in their ability to lift weights. Experience the power of gua-sha therapy and unlock your true potential in weightlifting.

Experience the ultimate relief for back pain in older adults with our revolutionary treatments. Choose between the rejuvenating gua-sha or the soothing hot pack, both of which have been proven to provide remarkable relief from symptoms. Say goodbye to discomfort and hello to a life free from back pain. Experience the long-lasting effects of gua-sha like never before. Experience the incredible benefits of gua-sha treatment! Just one week after receiving this amazing therapy, participants reported a remarkable increase in flexibility and a significant reduction in back pain. Don't miss out on the transformative effects of gua-sha - try it today!

Discover the Unforeseen Consequences and Potential Hazards

Experience the transformative power of Gua-sha as it delicately stimulates the capillaries, gently invigorating your skin's surface. Introducing a remarkable feature that leaves a lasting impression - a vibrant red or crimson bruise, famously known as the exquisite "sha". Experience the temporary discomfort of injuries that typically subside within a matter of days or weeks, leaving behind a gentle tenderness as they heal. Discover the perfect solution to your discomfort and bloating with an exceptional over-the-counter painkiller like Ibuprofen. Experience the relief you deserve and say goodbye to those pesky aches. Introducing the ultimate solution for safeguarding your precious bruised region! With our innovative product, you can now shield your delicate skin from any unwanted bumps. Stay cautious and keep your bruised area safe with our top-of-the-line protection. Discover the incredible benefits of applying a snowpack to alleviate swelling and bring much-needed relief to any discomfort you may be experiencing. Experience the soothing power of a snowpack today!

Experience the art of Gua-sha with utmost confidence as our skilled professionals delicately work their magic on your skin. Rest assured, our experts prioritize your safety and will never break your skin layer during the procedure. However, it's important to acknowledge that like any treatment, there are potential risks that could arise. Trust in our expertise and let us take care of your Gua-sha experience. Experience the ultimate in cleanliness and safety with our gua-sha specialists. We understand that even the smallest cut on the surface can increase the risk of illness. That's why our dedicated professionals go above and beyond, meticulously sterilizing their tools between each and every treatment. Trust us to prioritize your well-being and provide you with the highest standards of hygiene.

Discover the wonders of Gua-sha, a therapy that may not be suitable for everyone. If you fall into any of the following categories, it's best to avoid this treatment:

Introducing our exclusive solution for individuals with

skin or vein-related medical conditions. Say goodbye to worries about bleeding easily with our revolutionary product.

Introducing our exclusive solutions for two distinct groups of individuals:

• Individuals who prioritize their health by taking medication to effectively thin their blood.

• Individuals who have experienced deep vein thrombosis and are seeking effective solutions.

Introducing an exclusive opportunity for individuals who have encountered contamination, tumors, or wounds that have yet to fully heal.

Introducing a revolutionary feature for our valued customers: the option to seamlessly integrate with your existing implants, such as pacemakers or internal defibrillators. Experience the ultimate convenience and peace of mind with our cutting-edge technology.

Discover the Truth: Is Gua-sha Painful?

Discover the world of pain-free treatments! While traditional methods may cause discomfort, our revolutionary gua-sha technique deliberately induces bruising to unlock your body's natural healing powers. Rest assured, any temporary discomfort will fade away in just a few days, leaving you feeling rejuvenated and revitalized.

Discover the Art of Gua-sha: Unleash the Power of Gua-sha Tools and Master the Technique

Discover the Essential Equipment for Gua-Sha

Discover the incredible power of gua-sha, where a beautifully designed handheld tool with elegantly curved edges is expertly employed to unlock your body's natural healing potential. Introducing the latest innovation in skin care techniques! Say goodbye to traditional methods and embrace the modern approach. Our skilled therapists now utilize a sleek, hand-held tool with perfectly rounded edges, ensuring a gentle and precise experience. No more spoons or coins - it's time to elevate your skincare routine!

Introducing the revolutionary Gua-sha tools that are

expertly designed to provide the perfect balance of weight, allowing the specialist to effortlessly apply precise pressure. Say goodbye to the struggle and experience the ultimate ease with our innovative Gua-sha tools.

Discover the incredible power of Traditional East Asian Medication and its ability to support healing. Immerse yourself in the world of Bian rock, jade, and rose quartz, materials that are revered by professionals for their remarkable properties. Experience the superior quality of medical-grade stainless steel, the perfect choice for IASTM and gua-sha treatments in any medical setting. Experience the expertise of skilled professionals as they delicately apply a carefully measured amount of gas to the precise area of your body undergoing treatment. This ingenious technique enables the therapist to effortlessly glide their specialized tool over your skin, ensuring maximum efficiency and optimal results. Experience the art of gua-sha like never before with our skilled practitioner. Feel the gentle yet invigorating pressure of our specially designed devices as they glide smoothly and firmly along your body, following a single path. Discover the transformative power of gua-sha today. Experience the ultimate relaxation and rejuvenation with Gua-sha. To fully indulge in this ancient healing technique, simply lie face down on a luxurious massage therapy table while our skilled practitioners work their magic on your trunk or back of the legs. Prepare to be transported to a state of pure bliss and wellness.

Chapter 4

Introducing Gua-Sha: The Ultimate DIY Beauty Tool for Achieving a Radiant Glow from the Inside Out!

Discover the perfect harmony between self-care and skincare as Eva Ramirez delves into the ancient ritual of Gua-sha. Uncover the remarkable benefits it holds for both your overall well-being and radiant complexion.

Introducing Gua-sha (pronounced gwa-sha), the ancient self-care practice rooted in traditional Chinese medicine. Introducing the incredible power of a specialized tool, meticulously crafted from the finest jade, bone, or horn. Experience the transformative effects as this extraordinary tool gently glides across your skin, skillfully redirecting the flow of energy within your body. Witness as stagnant energy is effortlessly divided, leaving behind a sense of tranquility and reducing irritation. Prepare to be amazed as blood flow is invigorated, promoting a natural healing process within your body. Unlock the potential of your lymphatic system as it is stimulated, working harmoniously to restore balance and promote overall well-being. Embrace the ancient wisdom of this remarkable technique and embark on a journey of rejuvenation and self-discovery. Discover the incredible power of this time-tested technique that effortlessly tackles a wide range of issues. From soothing fevers and muscle pain to relieving pressure and swelling, this technique is your secret weapon against chronic coughs, sinusitis, and migraines.

Discover the transformative power of self-care, a cornerstone of Chinese Medicine known as Yang Sheng, meaning the art of living a healthy life. Experience the timeless tradition of Gua-sha, a cherished wellness ritual that has been passed down through generations. Originally practiced in the comfort of one's own home, this ancient technique has now gained widespread popularity in Western culture. Experience the rejuvenating power of Gua-sha massage therapy, a sought-after remedy offered by skilled acupuncturists and professionals in their state-of-the-art centers. Just like cupping or acupressure, Gua-sha massage therapy is designed to provide you with unparalleled relief and relaxation. Introducing the revolutionary prop-assisted athletic therapeutic massage! This cutting-edge technique is designed to reduce pressure and provide targeted relief to your neck, legs, and arms. Our skilled therapists will hone in on the areas that need attention, leaving you feeling rejuvenated and revitalized. Say goodbye to tension and hello to ultimate relaxation with our prop-assisted massage! Experience the power of our revolutionary treatment that harnesses the friction from each stroke to create a mesmerizing effect. Witness the captivating bruising and inflammation that may linger, leaving you in awe long after your session.

Discover the Benefits of Incorporating Dry Body Cleaning into Your Daily Routine!

Discover the fascinating connection between this and the world of beauty and skincare. Discover the transformative power of the gentler version of the Gua-sha technique, a true miracle for your facial skin. Discover the power of your regular everyday skincare routine - it's like having a personal therapist for your skin! Say goodbye to the need for expensive visits and let your skincare take care of your skin's health and well-being. Trust in the transformative benefits of your everyday routine.

Discover the Transformative Power of Reiki for Your Skin Layer!

Experience the incredible power of the Gua-sha tool with just a one-minute daily application. Witness the magic unfold as you enjoy instant results and unlock a world of long-term benefits for your well-being. Discover the incredible benefits of incorporating an everyday ritual into your skincare routine. Scientific studies have revealed that this simple practice can enhance microcirculation by an astounding 100%, resulting in reduced wrinkles, rejuvenated and toned skin, and a smoother complexion. Not only that, but it also boosts collagen production, effectively combating pigmentation, dark circles, and puffy eyes. Say goodbye to dullness and hello to defined jawlines as this ritual even helps decongest sinuses. Experience the transformative power of this ritual today!

Experience the sensation of gently caressing your way to radiant and rejuvenated skin. Our innovative formula penetrates deep beneath the surface, nourishing your skin from within. Not only will you achieve a healthy glow, but you'll also feel the tension melt away as it soothes your facial muscles, providing relief from nighttime jaw clenching. Experience the ultimate solution for soothing soreness, any day, with our incredibly sensible approach. Discover the incredible power of the Gua-sha! If you find yourself plagued by those pesky eye twitches caused by insomnia or stress, look no further. With just a gentle touch, the Gua-sha can work wonders in supporting, relieving, and relaxing your tired eye muscles. Say goodbye to those annoying twitches and hello to blissful relaxation!

Discover the ultimate tool for your beauty routine - the exquisite jade gua-sha. Ensure you have the perfect instrument to achieve flawless results with ease.

Introducing the exquisite green rock that not only adds a touch of beauty to your dresser, but also boasts remarkable air-con properties. Say goodbye to anything made from bone and horn for obvious reasons, and embrace the elegance of this revered gem. Discover the wisdom in steering clear of lower-priced alternatives that could potentially be crafted from acrylic or other synthetic chemicals that have the potential to cause irritation to your delicate skin. Experience the ultimate luxury of effortlessly gliding stones across your skin while simultaneously nourishing and moisturizing with our exquisite facial oil. Elevate your massage routine to new heights with the perfect combination of smoothness and hydration.

Introducing Katie Brindle, the extraordinary Chinese medicine specialist and visionary behind Hayo'u - a remarkable all-natural medical health insurance and skincare brand hailing from the illustrious U.K. Introducing Hayo'u - your gateway to the world of Chinese medication. We believe in making self-treatment easy and accessible through our simple daily rituals and useful techniques. Say goodbye to complicated methods and hello to a more approachable approach to wellness. Discover the exquisite equipment they have to offer, including their renowned Gua-sha. Meticulously carved from traditional Xiuyan Jade, this luxurious tool comes with a plush velvet pouch, making it perfect for your travels. Enhance your self-care routine with their collection of short, user-friendly videos, designed to help you master the art of the ritual in the comfort of your own home.

Experience the transformative power of weather practice, a refreshing ritual that can be embraced both in the tranquil moments of the morning and the serene moments of the evening. By incorporating this mindful beauty practice into your daily routine, you can effortlessly release the burdens of the day and restore a sense of calm and serenity to your visage. Prepare to embark on a meditative and rejuvenating journey that will leave you feeling relaxed and revitalized.

Discover the Art of Gua-sha: Master the

Technique for a Radiant Face in 11 Effortless Steps

Prepare to be amazed when I detect that you've probably experienced the wonders of a Gua-Sha treatment for your face and throat. Discover the captivating world of historical treatments, where the past comes alive in vivid detail. But wait, there's more! Introducing the all-new face version, a revolutionary twist that adds a whole new dimension to your experience. Prepare to be amazed!

Discover the Amazing Benefits of Face Gua-Sha

Introducing Gua-Sha, the ultimate secret to rejuvenating your facial skin and neck. Often referred to as the Eastern Botox or Eastern Facelift, this ancient technique is here to revolutionize your beauty routine. Introducing the incredible power of traditional Chinese Medication treatment for your facial skin. Experience the remarkable benefits it brings:

- Revitalize and rejuvenate your facial muscles with our exceptional support system.

- Experience the transformative power of our revolutionary skincare product. Our formula is specially designed to smooth and rejuvenate your skin, leaving it looking flawless and youthful. Say goodbye to pesky lines and wrinkles, and say hello to a radiant complexion. Try it today and see the incredible results for yourself.

- Discover the ultimate solution for those pesky dark circles and stubborn eyebags beneath your eyes. Say goodbye to the signs of aging with our revolutionary formula.

- Experience the power of our revolutionary formula that effectively lightens age and other skin discolorations. Say goodbye to uneven skin tone and hello to a brighter, more radiant complexion.

- Experience the transformation as your tone blossoms into a vibrant and radiant glow.

- Introducing our revolutionary solution that effectively targets and eliminates acne, rosacea, and other common skin conditions. Say goodbye to blemishes and hello to a flawless complexion with our advanced formula.

Prepare to be amazed by the incredible results of body Gua-Sha! As someone who has personally experienced everything on the list, I can confidently say that the last item is the only one I haven't tried. But let me tell you, even with my high expectations from previous positive encounters with body Gua-Sha, I was absolutely blown away by the remarkable improvements I saw on my face.

Experience the transformative power of Glutathione and Grape Seed. Discover the secret to a clear and radiant face with the ancient technique of face Gua-Sha. Witness the remarkable results that these supplements can bring, as your complexion glows with unparalleled clarity and radiance. Don't miss out on the benefits that only these extraordinary products can provide.

Discover the Magic: How it Works

Introducing Gua-Sha, the ancient practice that rejuvenates your body with its unique scraping movements. Experience the soothing sensation as a smooth-edged tool glides across your skin, leaving you feeling refreshed and revitalized. Discover the incredible challenge of enhancing petechial, reddish marks through the transformative power of a Gua-Sha therapy program.

Introducing Gua-Sha Scraping for a Radiant Face! Introducing Gua-Sha, the gentle yet powerful skincare technique that will revolutionize your beauty routine. With its unique scraping action, Gua-Sha activates the layers of your skin, effectively clearing away stagnant lymph and reducing puffiness. But that's not all - this incredible tool also releases toxins, unveiling a radiant and luminous complexion. And let's not forget about the amazing massaging action, which effortlessly relaxes tense muscles and helps diminish the appearance of wrinkles. Experience the transformative power of Gua-Sha today!

Discover the Art of Eastern Botox in Just 11 Simple Steps!

Introducing essential tips for beginners:

- Avoid exerting excessive pressure, unlike when

vigorously scrubbing the body. Unlock the secret to success by embracing the power of light-weight solutions. Experience unparalleled efficiency and effortless productivity. Choose wisely, choose light-weight. Discover the exquisite delicacy of your facial skin, a true testament to its unique nature compared to other areas of your body.

Introducing our revolutionary technique: lymph movement for a rejuvenated face! Experience the ultimate detoxification as we expertly eliminate toxins through the precise and remaining lymphatic ducts. Discover the captivating allure of the spaces nestled between your collarbones.

Experience the effortless elegance of our upward (light) scraping movements. Introducing our revolutionary solution: Say goodbye to sagging with our innovative approach. Experience the power of uplift as we eliminate any downward actions. Join us on our journey to defy gravity and embrace a lifted future. Experience the exceptional benefits of our revolutionary technique, where the only exception lies in the finished part, should you choose to indulge in the exquisite process of dumping in the meticulously highlighted lymphatic ducts.

Introducing the revolutionary Cosmetic Gua-Sha! Unlock the secrets to youthful and radiant skin with our beginner's guide. Discover the essential steps to take on your journey to beauty:

Introducing the Third Vision: Experience a heart-stirring stroke that starts from the depths of your eyebrows and extends all the way to your hairline. Experience the incredible power of this region to activate the process of curing.

Discover the secret to a more youthful appearance with our revolutionary technique. Effortlessly glide your fingertips from the lower forehead, tracing a path above your eyebrows and extending towards your temples. Experience the sensation of rejuvenation as you indulge in this luxurious self-care ritual.

Enhance your beauty routine with the exquisite gua-sha tool. Discover the art of sculpting your eyebrows to perfection by delicately scraping the area beneath your brow and above your eye, using the gentle curve of the tool. Elevate your self-care experience and unlock your true radiance. Discover the hidden beauty of the brow bone.

• Captivate your senses: Gently caress the area where those pesky under-eye bags tend to appear, beginning from the inner corner of your nose and gliding up towards your temple. Experience the transformative power of gently shifting the stagnant lymph from the depths of your facial skin, all the way up to the temple and effortlessly towards the hairline.

Enhance your beauty routine with a simple yet effective technique for your cheek area. Experience the transformative power of a sweeping movement that will leave your cheeks looking radiant and flawless. Experience the luxurious sensation as you glide along the medial side of your nose, effortlessly tracing the contours of your cheek, and then gracefully making your way back to the center of your ear.

Introducing Jaws: Experience the incredible benefits

once more as you gently sweep the lymph upwards towards your ears.

Discover the art of defining your chin with a graceful sweep that starts from the very core of your face, glides beneath your lower lip, and elegantly extends to your earlobes.

Discover the secret to a perfectly sculpted jawline with our revolutionary technique. Begin by gently gliding the tool from the soft area beneath your chin, all the way to the elegant curve underneath your ears. Unveil a more defined and chiseled look today!

Introducing the ultimate throat care technique: Harness the power of gentle energy to delicately scrape from your jaw and earlobes, all the way to the center of your collarbone. Experience the rejuvenating sensation like never before!

Experience the ultimate sweep of rejuvenation: Gather all the lymph that has been displaced from your facial skin and gracefully release it into the realm of lymphatic drainage. Glide your fingers along the central path of your forehead, just below the hairline, and continue the journey through your temples and ears until you reach the majestic destination of your throat and terminus area. Experience the power of regularity for a spotless outcome.

Chapter 5

Experience the Ultimate Gua-Sha Face Treatment in the Comfort of Your Own Home

Discover the incredible benefits of gua-sha!

Introducing Gua-sha, the ancient art that predates acupuncture. With its heart stroke design, it gently awakens the meridian lines, the very pathways of life force. By activating the body's innate healing abilities, Gua-sha is here to revolutionize your well-being. Introducing gua-sha, the ultimate skin rejuvenation technique. Experience the power of collagen creation as it revitalizes your skin layer. Sculpt and shade your facial contours, while allowing irritation to effortlessly drain away. Feel the freedom as your muscles release all tension, creating their own supportive paths for a truly radiant complexion. Experience the transformative power of our product as it works wonders on your skin. Witness the magic as blood flow is enhanced, delivering vital nutrients to areas that have long been deprived. Say goodbye to blockages and hello to radiant, rejuvenated skin.

Experience the transformative power of Gua-Sha as it goes beyond the surface, revitalizing your meridian lines. Experience the incredible benefits that organs like the belly, liver, spleen, center, and kidneys have to offer. Experience the transformative power of gua-sha tools as they effortlessly glide from your facial skin to your kidneys, unlocking their full potential.

Discover the Astonishing Advantages!

Introducing our revolutionary product that delivers a nutrient-rich and oxygenated bloodstream directly to your skin layer and tissues. Experience the power of nourishment and rejuvenation like never before.

Introducing our revolutionary system that effectively drains lymph liquid, a common carrier of toxins and waste, from your cells, leaving them thoroughly cleansed.

Introducing our revolutionary solution that will banish

wrinkles from your life. Say goodbye to those pesky lines and hello to a smoother, more youthful complexion. Experience the magic of wrinkle elimination like never before.

Experience the ultimate solution for sagging epidermis with our revolutionary treatment. Our powerful formula not only tightens your skin layer but also helps prevent future sagging. Say goodbye to droopy skin and hello to a firmer, more youthful complexion.

Introducing our revolutionary solution that effectively banishes those pesky dark circles around your eyes. Say goodbye to tired-looking eyes and hello to a refreshed and rejuvenated appearance.

Experience the ultimate liberation for your skin with our revolutionary solution that banishes shaded areas and hyper-pigmentation. Say goodbye to uneven skin tone and hello to a radiant complexion.

Illuminate your complexion with our revolutionary formula.

Experience the remarkable power of our product that dramatically extends the healing time of breakouts and acne. Experience the ultimate solution for all your epidermis issues.

Experience the incredible power to heal and provide relief for rosacea with our exceptional product.

Experience the incredible power of our product to enhance penetration. Unlock new levels of success with our unparalleled support.

Introducing Goodies TMJ Disorder and Migraine Relief!

Introducing the revolutionary alternative to shots and face-lift surgery! Say goodbye to invasive procedures and hello to a more youthful appearance. Whether you choose to use it in the comfort of your own home or seek treatments from a qualified practitioner, this solution is here to transform your beauty routine.

Discover the Art of Choosing the Perfect Gua-sha Tool!

Discover a stunning array of exquisite Gua-sha tools,

each meticulously crafted in a variety of captivating designs, sizes, and forms. Introducing a collection of extraordinary devices crafted from the finest pet bone and horn, as well as exquisite gemstones such as jade and rose quartz. Elevate your style with these unique and captivating pieces. Discover the elegance and versatility of Chinese soup spoons, a must-have for professionals in various fields. Introducing the versatile cup jar with its sleek and ergonomic design. It's not just for sipping your favorite beverages, but it can also be used in a pinch as a cover. With its curved and soft sides, it's the perfect multi-purpose solution for all your needs.

Discover the hottest trends of the moment: quartz and jade.

Introducing Jade: The Ultimate Source of Serenity, Purity, and Fertility

Experience the soothing power of rose quartz as it effortlessly brings tranquillity and restores harmony to the depths of your heart. Introducing the extraordinary stone of universal love, a true symbol of compassion and care. Experience the power of unconditional love with this remarkable gem.

Discovering the perfect gua-sha rock is akin to selecting a precious crystal or gemstone. Experience the satisfaction of hand-picking your selection (we highly recommend it). Embrace the allure, indulge in its essence, and savor the tactile sensation as it graces your fingertips. Discover which one captivates your attention – if the first one is shimmering a bit brighter for you than the rest, choose it!

Discover the Key Ingredient for an Enriching Practice Experience!

Discover the secret to achieving and maintaining a thriving and healthy body: regularity. Experience the ultimate nourishment for your body and mind with our carefully curated selection of refreshing water, rejuvenating sleep, wholesome meals, and invigorating movement. Discover the incredible benefits of incorporating regular gua-sha therapy into your routine. Prepare to be amazed by the transformative effects it can have on your well-being. Discover the secret to optimal well-being: finding balance. The body flourishes when we avoid extremes and instead embrace the harmonious middle ground. Unlock your true potential by nourishing your gut, the key to overall health and vitality.

Discover the incredible power of incorporating this practice into your daily routine. With a remarkable 20 liters of liquid circulating through your body each day (including three liters of lymph fluid), you'll be amazed at the support it provides to your overall well-being. Discover the invigorating power of gua-sha in your daily routine. While it may seem challenging at first, dedicating just a few minutes a week can make a remarkable difference. Embrace the active lifestyle you deserve, even if it's only two minutes at a time. Indulge in the exquisite moments of self-care that your body craves.

Experience the transformative power of pressure and purpose in your practice. Discover the art of the gentle touch as you explore the various levels of pressure. Experience the transformative power of the gua-sha rock as it glides effortlessly across your face, following precise and purposeful movements. Unlock the secrets to radiant and youthful skin with every sweep. Experience the power of a gentle touch as you assist the lymph liquid and engage your muscles with increased pressure. Discover how being bigger can make a difference. Introducing our revolutionary product that will revolutionize your life! Experience the ultimate in care and comfort with our innovative solution. Say goodbye to bruising and distress with our cutting-edge technology. Take control of your well-being and embrace a life free from discomfort. Trust in our product to deliver the results you deserve. Don't wait, try it today and discover a new level of peace and tranquility. Your body will thank you!

Discover the Ultimate Way to Prep Your Skin Layer!

Experience the ultimate in skincare luxury with a meticulous routine. Begin by ensuring your face and hands are impeccably clean, setting the stage for a truly transformative experience. Elevate your skincare ritual by incorporating a sublime hydrosol such as the exquisite

True Botanicals Renew Nutrient Mist, the invigorating OSEA Sea Vitamin Boost, or the enchanting Heritage Store Rose Water. Once your canvas is prepped, indulge in the nourishing embrace of a facial oil. Immerse yourself in the opulence of True Botanicals Renew Radiance Oil, the rejuvenating OSEA Undaria Argan Oil, or the captivating Shiva Rose face oil. Gently massage the oil onto your face and neck, allowing the essence to envelop your skin in a veil of pure bliss. To enhance the experience, glide your gua-sha tool effortlessly across your face, utilizing the residual oil on your hands to ensure a smooth and seamless glide. Begin your journey with a sense of purpose and tranquility, as you take in deep, rejuvenating breaths.

Discover the Art of Gua-sha: Unleash Your Inner Beauty

Experience the Ultimate Cleanse - Transform your skincare routine with our revolutionary method. Begin by delicately drying your facial skin with a pristine washcloth, ensuring a fresh canvas. Then, indulge in a lavish misting of our specially formulated solution, leaving your face feeling rejuvenated and invigorated. Introducing the incredible hydrosol, the perfect companion to unlock the full potential of your essential oil. Prepare to embark on a journey of deep nourishment and hydration as you apply this luxurious elixir to the layers of your skin that crave revitalization. Introducing the ultimate hygiene hack: the one-time-use washcloth! Say goodbye to reusing dirty cloths and hello to a fresh, clean start every time you step into the shower. With our innovative design, simply toss your used washcloth into the hamper and enjoy the peace of mind that comes with a pristine bathing experience. Upgrade your daily routine with our game-changing washcloth today! Discover the ultimate solution for banishing breakouts! Say goodbye to reusing cosmetic towels without cleaning. Your skin deserves the best care. Experience the transformative power of bacteria as it delicately graces your skin once more.

Experience the rejuvenating power of Facial - Gas with just 4-10 drops. Gently apply this luxurious gas to your facial skin and throat, starting from the forehead and moving down towards the lymph liquid, for a truly invigorating experience. Experience the invigorating power of our revolutionary formula, designed to stimulate motion in your epidermis and cells. Prepare yourself for the ultimate gua-sha experience with our exceptional prepping solution.

Experience the soothing warmth of the Gua-sha tool as you gently rub it between your hands. Experience the ultimate convenience with our innovative tool that not only lubricates itself, but also ensures a smooth application without leaving any marks on untouched areas of your skin. Say goodbye to uneven lines and hello to flawless results.

Experience the ultimate sensation as you delicately glide your fingertips along the contours of your guitar neck. And now, imagine the sheer bliss as you gently sweep across your Adam's apple, igniting a wave of pure pleasure that will awaken your REN collection like never before. Introducing the extraordinary REN route in Chinese medication! This remarkable pathway harnesses the body's precious yin energy, providing a protective shield for the stomach, chest, neck, mind, and face. Experience the power of ancient healing and unlock your body's natural potential with the REN route!

Experience the ultimate sensation as you effortlessly glide our innovative tool under your chin, from your guts all the way to your earlobe. Feel the smoothness and precision like never before. Experience the ultimate in skincare comfort with our revolutionary device. Gently cradle the delicate skin beneath your chin with the utmost care, using your additional thumb. Effortlessly glide the device towards your earlobes, reversing the signs of aging in the most luxurious way possible.

Experience the art of facial massage as you sweep gracefully from the centre of your chin, tracing the contours of your jawline. With a delicate touch, guide the motion towards your earlobes, even giving a gentle jiggle to stimulate the flow of liquid. Witness the magic as the liquid gracefully drains down your throat, making its way towards the lymph nodes nestled just above your collarbone.

Discover the transformative power of sweeping underneath your cheekbone – Experience the effortless efficiency of effortlessly collecting generous quantities of liquid that is commonly stored in this convenient location, and expertly directing it towards your hairline. Experience the delicate and precise art of effortlessly maneuvering your tool along the hairline.

Experience the sensation of a gentle sweep across your flawless cheekbones, effortlessly gliding towards the elegant frame of your hairline.

Experience the gentle sensation of sweeping under your eye, as if caressing the delicate area. Allow your attention to effortlessly glide towards the midline, where the muscles naturally align with this path. Feel the subtle flow of lymph, like tiny streams, gently moving downwards from the inner corner of your eye to the outer part. Discover the ultimate technique for achieving flawless results with gua-sha. Instead of simply sweeping from the outside, why not try the more traditional approach of starting from the inside edge and gently gliding towards the hairline? This tried-and-true method is guaranteed to elevate your gua-sha experience to new heights.

Enhance the allure of your eyebrows by expertly sweeping from the inner corner towards the hairline, or even further beyond the brow bone. As you gracefully sweep upwards, remember to work in small, precise sections, gently gliding along the eyebrow in three to five seamless motions.

Experience the transformative power of sweeping from the middle of your eyebrows, effortlessly gliding over your eyes and towards the elegant curve of your hairline. Discover the subtle nuances of your clairvoyance as it becomes more activated, allowing you to perceive the unseen with clarity and grace.

Experience the ultimate beauty transformation with this revolutionary technique. Mastered by none other than Britta Plug of Britta Beauty in the heart of NYC, this method will sweep through the centre from your forehead out to your hairline, leaving you with a flawless and radiant look. Introducing the revolutionary sweeping technique that will transform your hair routine! With a gentle touch that starts from the guts of your forehead, our method avoids the hairline and gracefully glides into your locks. It continues its journey behind the ears and down the throat, leaving you with a flawless and stunning look. Experience pure bliss with our heavenly product.

Indulge in a luxurious self-care ritual by gently caressing the other part of your face. Begin this rejuvenating journey by lavishing attention on your neck, and gracefully progress through each step with utmost care.

Experience a seamless glide - Once you've perfected the rest of your facial routine, effortlessly sweep down the neck to promote lasting drainage. Discover the secret to a perfectly sculpted jawline with our revolutionary tool. With precision and care, effortlessly glide the tool along your jawbone, creating a graceful contour that will leave everyone in awe. Experience the confidence that comes with a defined jawline, as you sweep down towards your collarbone, revealing a more refined and elegant you.

Unlock the power of practice with these essential ideas:

Introducing the ultimate sweeping technique for maximum results! Prepare to take your skills to the next level with our expert recommendation: sweep each area not just once, not twice, but a minimum of three times! And for those looking to truly master the art of sweeping, we dare you to go beyond and sweep up to an impressive ten times. Get ready to elevate your practice and achieve sweeping perfection like never before!

Discover the secret to flawless skin with these expert tips:

- Achieve optimal results by keeping your tool at a perfect 15-degree angle to your skin layer, rather than the standard 90-degree approach.

- Say goodbye to discomfort and irritation! When you feel your tool tugging or pulling, simply apply a touch more gas for a smoother glide.

- Get ready to experience a revolutionary product that will exceed all your expectations. Discover the joy of exploring various aspects and types of tools that perfectly complement your unique face. Discover the power of individuality - what resonates with you may be different from what you see on screen.

Discover the secret to unlocking your skin's true potential with Gua-sha! Find out the optimal frequency for practicing this ancient beauty ritual.

Discover the transformative power of gua-sha and elevate your self-care routine to new heights. By incorporating gua-sha into your daily regimen, you can unlock a world of rejuvenation and relaxation. But remember, self-care should never feel like a chore. Take breaks when needed and listen to your body's cues. Embrace the blissful balance of activity and rest.

Experience the sensation like never before.

Experience the ultimate relaxation with Gua-sha, a technique renowned for its soothing effects. Discover the perfect pressure and indulge in gentle, loving strokes that will leave you feeling truly pampered. Experience the sensation of gliding the gua-sha tool effortlessly across your skin, as smooth and delicate as a newborn's. Indulge in the luxurious feeling of pampering yourself with this exquisite beauty ritual.

Experience the exhilarating sensation of fluid movement - it's absolutely fantastic! Experience the sensation of your skin coming alive, as if it's returning and waking up. Experience the power of feminine energy by starting your medication on the left side. Embrace the nurturing qualities that this side represents and open yourself up to receiving the benefits of your treatment. Discover the remarkable phenomenon where the rest of the body ignites a powerful response in its most receptive part. Experience the incredible synergy that occurs when every part of your body is in perfect harmony.

Discover the extraordinary potential of Gua-sha!

Discover the secret to flawless skin with gua-sha, the ancient beauty ritual. However, it's important to note that if you've recently received injections, it's best to avoid this invigorating practice. Prioritize your skin's health and consult with a skincare professional before incorporating gua-sha into your routine. Experience the transformative power of Botox with a minimum two-week stay.

Discover the secret to flawless skin! While gua-sha is a powerful tool for enhancing your complexion, it's important to use it wisely. Avoid using gua-sha over cystic acne, pimples, and start lesions, as this could potentially irritate these delicate areas. However, fear not! Gua-sha can still work wonders for your skin during a breakout, offering a multitude of benefits. Embrace the transformative power of gua-sha and unlock your skin's true potential! Experience the incredible benefits of draining below the breakout, as it effortlessly propels toxins towards the lymph nodes. Unlock the power of your lymphatic system today!

Experience the mesmerizing rhythm of each heart stroke as it resonates within the confines of the same region, precisely ten times. Are you tired of constantly repeating the same sweeping motion? Beware, as this could lead to an overwhelming level of activation. Experience the power of our potent liquids. But beware, indulging in too much can leave you feeling a bit off balance, with detoxification symptoms like dizziness or flu-like sensations. So sip wisely and savor the benefits.

Chapter 6

Introducing the revolutionary solution for cellulite!

Discover the secret to banishing cellulite and achieving smooth, flawless skin! Cellulite tends to make its unwelcome appearance around the hips and thighs, targeting those yang meridians. But fear not, because the key to tackling this pesky problem lies in targeting the Gall Bladder. Say goodbye to cellulite and hello to confidence! Introducing the Small Yang Meridian, where the Qi in the Gall Bladder flows with a subtle grace, often displaying a gentle strength that sets it apart from the other yang meridians. Introducing cellulite, the culprit behind the unsightly dimpling of your skin. It occurs when subcutaneous fat protrudes into the dermis, resulting in a noticeable undulating junction between your skin and adipose cells.

Introducing the incredible Spleen - the unsung hero that not only nourishes muscle and fat, but also plays a vital role in distributing fat evenly throughout your entire body, with a special focus on the periphery. Say hello to a harmonious physique like never before! Introducing the fascinating world of cellulite! Prepare to be amazed as we delve into the intricate workings of excess fat distribution. Picture this: fat that seems to mysteriously stagnate without proper circulation in specific regions of your body. It's like a captivating dance of biology! Introducing the undeniable truth: excess fat and poor circulation go hand in hand. Experience the captivating image of imbalance described earlier.

Introducing a fascinating dilemma that arises along the meridian of the body. This captivating issue can manifest itself in various forms, such as the Gall Bladder, Urinary Bladder, or even the Stomach, depending on the unique circumstances of each patient. Discover the key to optimal well-being by achieving perfect harmony between your Spleen and the affected meridians.

Introducing our revolutionary Body Acupuncture Treatment!

Say goodbye to cellulite around the lateral part of your

thighs with our cutting-edge solution. Experience the transformative power of acupuncture like never before.

Introducing the powerful duo for gall bladder health: UB 19, also known as the Back-Shu stage, and GB 37, the Luo level. Experience the ultimate support for your gall bladder with these two acupressure points.

Introducing the perfect solution for your spleen health - UB 20 (Back-Shu period) and St 40 (Luo place). Experience the incredible benefits today!

Introducing our exclusive local needles and moving cup massage! Experience the ultimate relaxation and rejuvenation with this unique therapy. With two sessions per week, you'll be on your way to total bliss. Don't miss out - book your 8-10 sessions today!

Unlock the power of this revolutionary treatment principle, available to all those affected by meridian in Atlanta. Introducing the incredible Bladder meridian! Unlock its full potential with the power duo of UB 28, the Back-Shu position, to enhance its function, and UB 58, the Luo-connecting point of the yang meridian, to invigorate the yang and diminish the yin aspect. Experience the remarkable benefits today!

Discover the incredible benefits of local treatment when it is executed with utmost precision and expertise. Discover the art of cupping massage therapy and embrace the journey towards wellness. While it may not always be a blissful experience, it's important to approach the process with patience and allow the healing to unfold naturally. Trust in the power of this ancient technique and let it work its magic at its own pace.

Introducing the Extraordinary Local Therapy Experience!

Experience the ultimate healing with our revolutionary treatment. For those seeking relief along the Gall Bladder meridian, we have a unique approach that will leave you feeling rejuvenated. Our expert therapists will guide you through a two-part session, ensuring maximum results. Lie down and indulge in the first half of the treatment, where tiny needles and cupping techniques will work their magic. Then, seamlessly transition to the other side for the same exceptional care. Discover the power of balance and harmony with our exclusive approach.

Discover the incredible power of lying privately and its impact on your body. Unlock the potential of UB 18, UB 20, St 40, and GB 37 acupressure points to enhance your well-being.

Introducing the all-new and improved. Get ready to experience a revolutionary product that will exceed all your expectations. Experience the revolutionary cellulite treatment that targets those stubborn areas with precision. Our expert technicians use a series of 10 to 15 local tiny needles, each measuring 15-20 cm in length and 0.20 mm in gauge. These needles are skillfully inserted perpendicularly, ensuring maximum effectiveness. With a distance of approximately 3 cm between each insertion, our technique is designed to deliver exceptional results.

Experience the ultimate relaxation with our body needles and local needles, expertly designed to provide maximum comfort and effectiveness. Leave them in your body for a blissful 20 minutes, allowing the healing powers to work their magic.

Experience the ultimate cellulite solution! Once those pesky needles are gone, it's time to indulge in the luxurious St John's wort oil. Gently apply this miracle elixir to the targeted cellulite area and watch it work its magic. Experience the ultimate relaxation of a massage therapy without any unnecessary friction. Remember, less is more when it comes to achieving the perfect balance.

Introducing our revolutionary cellulite glass! Experience the power of vacuum pressure as you place our specially designed cup on the reduced end of your thigh. Watch as the open fire creates a mesmerizing effect, while the cup effortlessly glides along your skin, leaving it beautifully red and rejuvenated. Experience the ultimate discomfort with this technique that is sure to leave the average person feeling less than satisfied. Don't let soreness hold you back - unleash the power of your vacuum and watch it reach new levels of efficiency. Experience the rejuvenating power of our massage therapy in just a minute.

Experience the incredible sensation of weightlessness in your legs after our rejuvenating treatment.

Introducing our revolutionary treatment plan, designed to be administered twice regularly, for a total of 8-10 sessions. Experience the power of our carefully crafted course, tailored to deliver exceptional results.

Discover the endless possibilities of what an average person can achieve in the comfort of their own home!

Discover the secret to banishing cellulite and enhancing circulation with a range of effective at-home techniques. Say goodbye to fat stagnation as you take control of your body's appearance.

Introducing the all-new and improved. This revolutionary product is here to change the game. Get ready to experience, Discover the culprits behind unwanted fat tissue in your body. Indulging in fatty foods and excessive consumption of fatty dairy products (remember, moderation is key for low-fat options) can contribute to the accumulation of fat. Additionally, be cautious of processed sugars, as they can also play a role. However, fear not! Wholemeal products, fruits, natural sugars, and honey can still be enjoyed guilt-free. Avoid these types of food at all costs!

Introducing the all-new and improved. This revolutionary product is here to change the game and exceed all your expectations Experience the transformative effects of reducing fat tissue thickness and improving blood flow. Discover the secret to a healthier lifestyle: staying hydrated with clean water. Make it a priority to drink water regularly throughout the day. Remember, it's not just about the quantity, but the consistency that matters. Stay refreshed and revitalized with every sip! Experience the incredible power of hot water as it effortlessly outperforms its cool counterpart. Witness the impressive speed at which patients delight in the soothing warmth of hot water. Discover a whole new level of satisfaction with hot water. Introducing the ultimate solution to combat cellulite! Say goodbye to those stubborn dimples with our revolutionary daily massage technique. Our specially designed soft spiky toners will gently caress your skin, while effectively breaking down stagnation in those trouble areas. Embrace a smoother, more toned appearance with our innovative approach to cellulite reduction. Experience the ultimate cellulite-busting sensation with our revolutionary seated cross-legged floor movement technique. By effortlessly gliding sideways, forwards, and backwards, you'll activate friction on those troublesome cellulite areas, giving you the confidence you deserve. Just 15 minutes a day in the comfort of your own home is all it takes to enhance blood flow and unlock radiant skin.

Experience the transformative power of Gua-sha Massage Therapy for cellulite in Singapore.

Are you tired of dealing with the unsightly, uneven texture of your skin on your hips, thighs, or buttocks? Experience the transformative power of Gua-sha Massage therapy for cellulite. Discover a world of rejuvenation and self-care with our comprehensive range of products. Embrace your true beauty without any shame or hesitation. Introducing Gua-Sha: Unveiling the Ancient Beauty Secret Introducing The Cellulite Remover: Your Solution for Smooth, Beautiful Skin!

Introducing Gua-Sha massage therapy, the ultimate solution for a wide range of ailments. Say goodbye to pains and aches, strains, lumbar stress, arthritis rheumatoid, and even heat stroke. Experience the transformative power of Gua-Sha today! Experience the incredible power of blood flow activation, unlocking its therapeutic impact and providing relief from the stagnation of your bloodstream.

Introducing the incredible Gua-sha Massage Cellulite! Say goodbye to cellulite with this revolutionary treatment that eliminates or reduces the appearance of cellulite in your body.

Experience the incredible advantages of Gua-Sha: • Enhance your skin's hydration levels for a radiant glow. • Say goodbye to stress as Gua-Sha melts away tension and promotes relaxation. • Achieve smoother, cellulite-free skin with the power of Gua-Sha. • Unwind and rejuvenate your face muscles, leaving you feeling refreshed and revitalized. • Boost your circulation and promote a healthier complexion with Gua-Sha's ability to improve blood flow. Discover the transformative benefits of Gua-Sha today!

Experience the transformative power of Gua-sha Massage Therapy:

Experience the transformative power of our Gua-Sha device on your oily skin. With gentle scraping motions, it effectively breaks down surface adhesion, boosts circulation, and improves lymph drainage. The result? Enhanced firmness and a radiant complexion. Introducing our revolutionary solution that not only tackles stubborn fat cells, but also promotes a flawlessly smooth and beautiful appearance.

Experience the incredible benefits of Gua-Sha, a rejuvenating technique that can be performed on any area of your body. Experience the transformative power of our services as we cater to every inch of your body, including the delicate canvas of your facial skin. Experience the ultimate skin rejuvenation with our revolutionary product. Discover the power of relaxation as it effortlessly enhances blood circulation and stimulates collagen production. Witness the transformation as your skin becomes radiant and youthful, bidding farewell to those pesky wrinkles. Elevate your skincare routine to new heights.

Discover the incredible power of massage techniques and dry brushing to effectively banish cellulite. Experience the incredible benefits of manually triggering your cells, enhancing blood flow and reducing unwanted tissues. Say goodbye to excess weight and hello to renewed energy. Experience the ultimate boost in skin radiance with our revolutionary product.

Acknowledgements

Behold the magnificent triumph of this extraordinary book, a testament to the divine intervention of God Almighty and the unwavering love and support of my cherished Family, devoted Fans, avid Readers, loyal Customers, and dear Friends. Their ceaseless encouragement has paved the way for this resounding success.

www.ingramcontent.com/pod-product-compliance
Lightning Source LLC
Chambersburg PA
CBHW031130020426
42333CB00012B/312